The Big Air Fryer Cookbook for weight loss

A Comprehensive Guide To Easy And Amazing Frying Recipes To Enjoy Your Time At Home.

Michael Blaze

Table of Contents

INTRODUCTION **8**

CHAPTER 1 BREAKFAST **10**

    1.   CHICKEN AND POTATO NUGGETS 10

    2.   HERBED SWEET POTATO HASH 14

    3.   SPINACH FRITTATA WITH CHERRY TOMATO 17

    4.   HERBED SALMON AND CHEESE FRITTATA 20

CHAPTER 2 SNACKS **24**

    5.   . SPICY CHICKPEAS 24

    6.   CRISPY CAULIFLOWER FLORETS 26

    7.   CLASSIC FRENCH FRIES 28

    8.   POTATO CHIPS IN OLIVE OIL 32

    9.   PARMESAN BREADED ZUCCHINI CHIPS 35

    10.   LOW-CARB CHEESE-STUFFED JALAPEÑO POPPERS 39

CHAPTER 3 BEEF & LAMB **42**

    11.   MOM'S SKIRT STEAK 42

    12.   TRADITIONAL FRENCH CHATEAUBRIAND 44

    13.   MONTREAL RIBEYE STEAK 46

    14.   ITALIAN RUMP ROAST 48

    15.   TENDERLOIN STEAKS WITH MUSHROOMS 50

CHAPTER 4 PORK..**52**

16.   CHEESEBURGER EGG ROLLS..52

17.   COPYCAT TACO BELL CRUNCH WRAPS.............................55

18.   COUNTRY FRIED STEAK..57

19.   TORTILLA ALA PORK...60

20.   PANKO-BREADED PORK CHOPS...62

CHAPTER 5 POULTRY..**66**

21.   MEXICAN CHICKEN...66

22.   HONEY DUCK BREASTS...68

23.   ROASTED CHICKEN AND VEGETABLE SALAD 70

24.   LEMON CHICKEN AND SPINACH SALAD 73

25.   ALMOND-CRUSTED CHICKEN NUGGETS.............................76

26.   EASY TANDOORI CHICKEN 79

CHAPTER 6 FISH & SEAFOOD..**82**

27.   CRAB CAKES WITH BELL PEPPERS.......................................82

28.   CRAB CAKES WITH LETTUCE AND APPLE SALAD...............85

29.   CRAB CAKES WITH SRIRACHA MAYONNAISE 89

30.   CRAB RATATOUILLE WITH EGGPLANT AND TOMATOES...........93

31.   CRAWFISH CREOLE CASSEROLE..96

32.   CRAB CAKES 99

33.   COCONUT SHRIMP 101

CHAPTER 7 VEGETABLES **104**

34.   INDIAN TURNIPS SALAD...104

35.   SPINACH PIE 107

36.   BEETS AND BLUE CHEESE SALAD 110

CHAPTER 8 SIDE DISH **112**

37.   BRUSSELS SPROUTS SIDE DISH...112

38.   HERBED POTATOES 114

CHAPTER 9 APPETIZERS **117**

39.   ITALIAN SHRIMP PLATTER 117

40.   POTATO CHIPS IN CHILI..119

CONCLUSION **121**

Introduction

Hi, first of all I have a challenge for you.

I ask you to leave a review by posting an image of a dish cooked using this cookbook, this would be a very nice and useful thing. Can you cook like Brandon?

Nothing is quite as satisfying as the sound of a crisp, savory fry coming out of the skillet. Some people will argue that french fries are simply not complete without ketchup, while others prefer to drench their crispy fried potatoes in honey or homemade mayonnaise.

In recent years, an alternative cooking technique has emerged in kitchens all across America. Gone are the days when frying food required constant attention and a deep fryer full of sizzling oil. Air frying, a combination of existing technology and good old-fashioned culinary know-how, has taken chefs and cooks by storm.

Air fryers use an air circulation technology to trap the heat produced by a heating element. The heat is then distributed around the food being cooked, cooking it from all sides at once. This means no more standing around for hours, waiting for a pot of oil to get hot enough to cook your favorite dishes!

Chapter 1 Breakfast

1. Chicken and Potato Nuggets

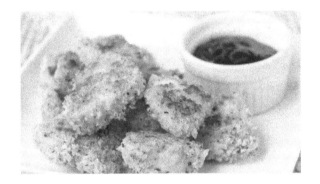

Preparation Time: 10 minutes

Cooking Time: 12 minutes

Servings: 3

Ingredients:

- 1 lb. minced chicken breast

- olive oil spray

- fillet

For the breading:

- 1 c. mashed potato

- 2 beaten eggs

- 1 egg

- ¾ c. breadcrumbs

- salt and pepper

Directions:

1. Combine chicken, mashed potato, and egg in a mixing bowl. Season with salt and pepper to taste. Spoon about 1 ½ tablespoon of mixture and form into 1-

inch thick bite-sized pieces (nuggets). Place in a large platter. Set aside as you prepare the breading ingredients.

2. In a mixing bowl, place breadcrumbs and season with salt and pepper.

3. Place seasoned breadcrumbs and eggs in separate bowls.

4. Coat each chicken and potato nugget with beaten eggs, and then in breadcrumbs.

5. Preheat your Air Fryer to 390°F.

6. Place chicken and potato nuggets in the cooking basket. Spray with oil. Do not overcrowd to have an equal distribution of heat while cooking.

7. Cook for about 7-10 minutes, or until golden brown.

8. Serve and enjoy!

Nutrition: Calories: 271 Fat: 12.2 g. Carbs: 16.1 g. Protein:

24.2 g.

2. Herbed Sweet Potato Hash

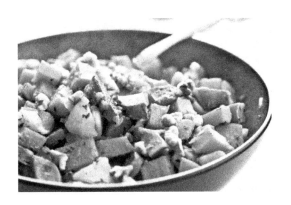

Preparation Time: 10 minutes

Cooking Time: 20 minutes

Servings: 3

Ingredients:

- 4 sweet potatoes, peeled and

- 1 c. sliced button mushrooms

- 1 chopped onion

- ½ chopped green bell pepper

- 2 tbsps. lemon juice

- 2 tbsps. olive oil

- ½ tsp. thyme, dried

- ½ tsp. rosemary, dried

- salt, and pepper

Directions:

1. Preheat Air Fryer to 360°F.

2. In a mixing bowl, mix together all ingredients. Season with salt and diced pepper.

3. Take out Air Fryer cooking basket, and then place sweet potato mixture.

4. Cook for about 25-30 minutes.

5. Serve and enjoy!

Nutrition: Calories: 203 Fat: 6.5 g. Carbs: 36.2 g. Protein: 3.4 g.

3. Spinach Frittata with Cherry Tomato

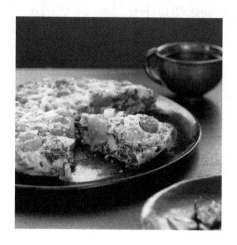

Preparation Time: 10 minutes

Cooking Time: 15 minutes

Servings: 2

Ingredients:

- 6 eggs

- kosher salt

- ground black pepper

- 2 tbsps. olive oil

- 1 chopped onion

- 1 c. halved cherry tomatoes

- 8 oz. spinach leaves

- 3 oz. grated cheddar

Directions:

1. Preheat oven to 390°F.

2. In a mixing bowl, whisk 6 eggs together and season with salt and pepper to taste. Set aside.

3. Set a skillet over medium-high heat and heat olive oil. Stir-fry the onion for 3 minutes, then add the spinach

leaves and cherry tomatoes. Cook for 3 minutes, stirring often.

4. Transfer vegetables to a small baking pan (enough to fit Air Fryer), pour the beaten eggs. Sprinkle with cheddar cheese.

5. Place baking pan in the Air Fryer cooking basket and cook for about 10 minutes.

6. Serve and enjoy!

Nutrition: Calories: 215 Fat: 12.9 g. Carbs: 8.5 g. Protein: 14.2 g.

4. Herbed Salmon and Cheese Frittata

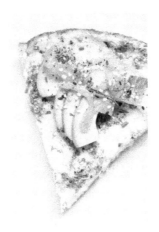

Preparation Time: 10 minutes

Cooking Time: 15 minutes

Servings: 3

Ingredients:

- 6 eggs

- kosher salt

- ground black pepper

- 2 tbsps. olive oil

- 1 chopped white onion

- 1 minced garlic clove

- 8 oz. baked salmon, diced

- 2 tbsps. freshly chopped dill

- 2 oz. grated cheddar

- 2 tbsps. chopped parsley

Directions:

1. Preheat oven to 390°F.

2. In a mixing bowl, whisk 6 eggs together and season with salt and pepper to taste.

3. Heat olive oil in a skillet over medium Sheat. Stir-fry onion and garlic for 3 minutes. Add the salmon and dill; cook further 2-3 minutes.

4. Transfer mixture in a small baking dish (enough to fit the Air Fryer cooking basket), pour the beaten egg mixture. Sprinkle with cheddar cheesweed.

5. Place baking dish in the Air Fryer cooking basket and cook for about 10 minutes.

6. Transfer into a baking dish and sprinkle with chopped parsley.

7. Serve and enjoy!

Nutrition: Calories: 217 Fat: 12.5 g. Carbs: 4.7 g. Protein: 18.8 g.

Chapter 2 Snacks

5. . Spicy Chickpeas

Preparation Time: 15 minutes

Cooking Time: 12 minutes

Servings: 4

Ingredients:

- 14 oz. can of chickpeas, rinsed, drained, and pat dry

- ½ tsp. chili powder

- 1 tbsp. olive oil

- Pepper

- Salt

Directions:

1. Place the air fryer Basket onto the Baking Pan and spray with cooking spray. Add chickpeas, chili powder, oil, pepper, and salt into the bowl and toss well. Spread chickpeas on an air fryer basket. Set to air fry at 375°F for 12 minutes. Serve and enjoy!

Nutrition: Calories: 192 Fat: 6 g. Fiber: 9 g. Carbs: 12 g. Protein: 3 g.

6. Crispy Cauliflower Florets

Preparation Time: 15 minutes

Cooking Time: 20 minutes

Servings: 4

Ingredients:

- 5 cups cauliflower florets

- 4 tbsps. olive oil

- ½ tsp. cumin powder

- 6 garlic cloves, chopped tsp. salt

Directions:

1. Put the air fryer basket onto the baking ban and spray using cooking spray. Add all the fixing into the large

bowl and toss well. Put cauliflower florets into the air fryer basket. Air fry at 400°F for 20 minutes. Serve and enjoy!

Nutrition: Calories: 192 Fat: 6 g. Fiber: 9 g. Carbs: 12 g. Protein: 3 g.

7. Classic French Fries

Preparation Time: 5 minutes

Cooking Time: 30 minutes

Servings: 6

Ingredients:

- 3 large russet potatoes

- 1 tbsp. canola oil

- 1 tbsp. extra-virgin olive oil

- Salt Pepper

Directions:

1. Peel the potatoes and cut lengthwise to create French

   fries.

2. Place the potatoes in a large bowl of cold water. Allow the potatoes to soak in the water for at least 30 minutes, preferably an hour. (See Prep tip.)

3. Spread the fries onto a baking sheet (optional: lined with parchment paper) and coat them with canola oil, olive oil, and salt and pepper to taste.

4. Transfer half of the fries to the air fryer basket. Cook for 10 minutes.

5. Open the air fryer and shake the basket so that the fries that were at the bottom come up to the top. Cook for an additional 5 minutes.

6. When the first half finishes, remove the cooked fries, then repeat steps 4 and 5 for the remaining fries.

7. Cool before serving.

Prep tip: Soaking the potatoes in water will remove the excess starch from the potatoes. This results in crispy, crunchy fries. If you do not soak the potatoes first, they will likely turn out soft. You can prep and soak the potatoes in advance of cooking—for weeknight dinners, I do this while I prepare the main course.

Cooking tip: Use your judgment and overall preference to determine how long the fries should cook. If the fries need to be crisper, allow them to cook for additional time. Really crisp fries may need to cook for up to 20 minutes. Some of this may also depend on how thick you cut the potatoes.

Nutrition: Calories: 168 Total fat: 5 g. Saturated fat: 1 g.

Cholesterol: 0 mg. Sodium: 38 mg. Carbohydrates: 29 g.

Fiber: 4 g. Protein: 3 g.

8. Potato Chips in Olive Oil

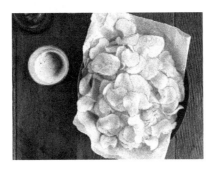

Preparation: 10 minutes **Cooking:** 30 minutes **Servings:** 5

Ingredients:

- 3 sweet potatoes 2 tsps. extra-virgin olive oil

- 1 tsp. cinnamon (optional) Salt Pepper

Directions:

1. Peel the sweet potatoes using a vegetable peeler. Cut the potatoes crosswise into thin slices. You can also use a mandoline to slice the potatoes into chips.

2. Place the sweet potatoes in a large bowl of cold water for 30 minutes. This helps remove the starch from the sweet potatoes, which promotes crisping.

3. Drain the sweet potatoes. Dry the slices thoroughly with paper towels or napkins.

4. Place the sweet potatoes in another large bowl. Drizzle with the olive oil and sprinkle with the cinnamon, if using, and salt and pepper to taste. Toss to fully coat.

5. Place the sweet potato slices in the air fryer. It is okay to stack them, but do not overcrowd. You may need to cook the chips in two batches. Cook the potatoes for 10 minutes.

6. Open the air fryer and shake the basket. Cook the chips for an additional 10 minutes.

7. Cool before serving.

Cooking tip: Before removing all of the chips from the air fryer, test one to ensure it is crunchy and has finished cooking.

Nutrition: Calories: 94 Total fat: 2 g. Saturated fat: 0 g. Cholesterol: 0 mg. Sodium: 58 mg. Carbohydrates: 20 g. Fiber: 2 g. Protein: 1 g.

9. Parmesan Breaded Zucchini Chips

Preparation Time: 15 minutes

Cooking Time: 20 minutes

Servings: 5

Ingredients:

For the zucchini chips:

- 2 medium zucchini

- 2 eggs

- 1/3 cup bread crumbs

- 1/3 cup grated Parmesan cheese

- Salt

- Pepper

- Cooking oil

For the lemon aioli:

- ½ cup mayonnaise

- ½ tbsp. olive oil

- Juice of ½ lemon

- 1 tsp. minced garlic

- Salt

- Pepper

Directions:

To make the zucchini chips

1. Slice the zucchini into thin chips (about 1/8 inch thick) using a knife or mandoline.

2. In a small bowl, beat the eggs. In another small bowl, combine the bread crumbs, Parmesan cheese, and salt and pepper to taste.

3. Spray the air fryer basket with cooking oil.

4. Dip the zucchini slices one at a time in the eggs and then the bread crumb mixture. You can also sprinkle the bread crumbs onto the zucchini slices with a spoon.

5. Place the zucchini chips in the air fryer basket, but do not stack. Cook in batches. Spray the chips with cooking oil from a distance (otherwise, the breading may fly off). Cook for 10 minutes.

6. Remove the cooked zucchini chips from the air fryer, then repeat step 5 with the remaining zucchini.

To make the lemon aioli

1. While the zucchini is cooking, combine the mayonnaise, olive oil, lemon juice, and garlic in a small bowl, adding salt and pepper to taste. Mix well until fully combined.

2. Cool the zucchini and serve alongside the aioli.

Cooking tip: Check-in on the zucchini chips throughout the cooking process to monitor doneness and adjust cook time as necessary. The zucchini will turn deep golden brown when crisp.

Nutrition: Calories: 192 Total fat: 13 g. Saturated fat: 3 g. Cholesterol: 97 mg. Sodium: 254 mg. Carbohydrates: 12 g. Fiber: 4 g. Protein: 6 g.

10. Low-Carb Cheese-Stuffed Jalapeño Poppers

Preparation: 10 minutes **Cooking Time:** 5 minutes

Servings: 5

Ingredients:

- 10 jalapeño peppers

- 6 oz. cream cheese

- ¼ cup shredded Cheddar cheese

- 2 tbsps. panko bread crumbs Cooking oil

Directions:

1. I recommend you wear gloves while handling jalapeños. Halve the jalapeños lengthwise. Remove

the seeds and the white membrane. (Save these if you

prefer spicy poppers; see Variation tip.)

2. Place the cream cheese in a small, microwave-safe

    bowl. Microwave for 15 seconds to soften.

3. Remove the bowl from the microwave. Add the

    Cheddar cheese. Mix well.

4. Stuff each of the jalapeño halves with the cheese

    mixture, then sprinkle the panko bread crumbs on

    top of each popper.

5. Place the poppers in the air fryer. Spray them with

    cooking oil. Cook for 5 minutes.

6. Cool before serving.

Substitution tip: Want to save some calories? Opt for reduced-fat cream cheese.

Variation tip: If you prefer five-alarm poppers, reserve the seeds and membrane when cutting the jalapeños in step 1, and add them to the cheese mixture in step 3.

Nutrition: Calories: 156 Total fat: 14 g. Saturated fat: 9 g. Cholesterol: 43 mg. Sodium: 874 mg. Carbohydrates: 3 g. Fiber: 1 g. Protein: 4 g.

Chapter 3 Beef & Lamb

11. Mom's Skirt Steak

Preparation Time: 10 minutes

Cooking Time: 15 minutes

Servings: 4

Ingredients:

- 1 ½ lbs. skirt steak

- Kosher salt and freshly cracked black pepper, to taste

- 1 tsp. cayenne pepper

- ¼ tsp. cumin powder

- 2 tbsps. olive oil

- 2 garlic cloves, minced

Directions:

1. Toss the steak with the other ingredients; place the steak in the Air Fryer cooking basket.

2. Cook the steak at 400°F for 12 minutes, turning it over halfway through the cooking time.

3. Bon appétit!

Nutrition: Calories: 305 Fat: 17.5 g. Carbs: 1.8 g. Protein: 35.2 g. Sugars: 0.6 g. Fiber: 0.3 g.

12. Traditional French Chateaubriand

Preparation: 10 minutes **Cooking Time:** 15 minutes

Servings: 4

Ingredients:

- 1 lb. beef filet mignon

- Sea salt and ground black pepper, to taste

- 1 tsp. cayenne pepper 3 tbsps. olive oil

- 1 tbsp. Dijon mustard

- 4 tbsps. dry French wine

Directions:

1. Toss the filet mignon with the rest of the ingredients;

   place the filet mignon in the Air Fryer cooking basket.

2. Cook the filet mignon at 400°F for 14 minutes, turning it over halfway through the cooking time.

3. Enjoy!

Nutrition: Calories: 249 Fat: 15.5 g. Carbs: 1.8 g. Protein: 26.2 g. Sugars: 0.8 g. Fiber: 0.4 g.

13. Montreal Ribeye Steak

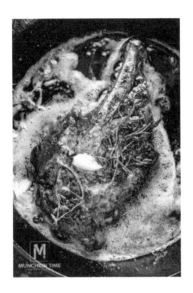

Preparation Time: 10 minutes

Cooking Time: 20 minutes

Servings: 4

Ingredients:

- 1 ½ lbs. ribeye steak, bone-in

- 2 tbsps. butter

- 1 Montreal seasoning mix

- Sea salt and ground black pepper, to taste

Directions:

1. Toss the ribeye steak with the remaining ingredients; place the ribeye steak in a lightly oiled Air Fryer cooking basket.

2. Cook the ribeye steak at 400°F for 15 minutes, turning it over halfway through the cooking time.

3. Bon appétit!

Nutrition: 357 Calories; 23.5g Fat; 2.7g Carbs; 33.5g Protein; 0.2g Sugars; 0.4g Fiber

14. Italian Rump Roast

Preparation Time: 10 minutes

Cooking Time: 55 minutes

Servings: 4

Ingredients:

- 1 ½ lbs. rump roast

- 2 tbsps. olive oil

- Sea salt and ground black pepper, to taste

- 1 tsp. Italian seasoning mix

- 1 onion, sliced

- 2 garlic cloves, peeled

- ¼ cup red wine

Directions:

1. Toss the rump roast with the rest of the ingredients; place the rump roast in a lightly oiled Air Fryer cooking basket.

2. Cook the rump roast at 390°F for 55 minutes, turning it over halfway through the cooking time.

3. Bon appétit!

Nutrition: 297 Calories; 16.9g Fat; 0.7g Carbs; 35.2g Protein; 0.2g Sugars; 0.1g Fiber

15. Tenderloin Steaks with Mushrooms

Preparation Time: 10 minutes

Cooking Time: 20 minutes

Servings: 4

Ingredients:

- 1 ½ lbs. tenderloin steaks

- 2 tbsps. butter, melted

- 1 tsp. garlic powder

- ½ tsp. mustard powder

- 1 tsp. cayenne pepper

- Sea salt and ground black pepper, to taste

- ½ lb. cremini mushrooms, sliced

Directions:

1. Toss the beef with 1 tablespoon of the butter and spices; place the beef in the Air Fryer cooking basket.

2. Cook the beef at 400°F for 10 minutes, turning it over halfway through the cooking time.

3. Add in the mushrooms along with the remaining 1 tablespoon of the butter. Continue to cook for an additional 5 minutes. Serve warm.

4. Bon appétit!

Nutrition: 310 Calories; 17g Fat; 3.7g Carbs; 41.2g Protein; 1.6g Sugars; 1.7g Fiber

Chapter 4 Pork

16. Cheeseburger Egg Rolls

Preparation Time: 15 minutes

Cooking Time: 10 minutes

Servings: 6

Ingredients:

- 6 eggs roll wrappers

- 6 chopped dill pickle chips

- 1 tbsp. yellow mustard

- 3 tbsps. cream cheese

- 3 tbsps. shredded cheddar cheese

- ½ c. chopped onion

- ½ c. chopped bell pepper

- ¼ tsp. onion powder

- ¼ tsp. garlic powder

- 8 oz. of raw lean ground beef

Directions:

1. In a skillet, add seasonings, beef, onion, and bell pepper. Stir and crumble beef till fully cooked, and vegetables are soft.

2. Take the skillet off the heat and add cream cheese, mustard, and cheddar cheese, stirring till melted.

3. Pour beef mixture into a bowl and fold in pickles.

4. Lay out egg wrappers and place 1/6th of beef mixture into each one. Moisten egg roll wrapper edges with water. Fold sides to the middle and seal with water.

5. Repeat with all other egg rolls.

6. Place rolls into air fryer, one batch at a time. Cook 7-9 minutes at 392°F.

Nutrition: Calories: 153 Fat: 4g Protein: 12g Sugar: 3g

17. Copycat Taco Bell Crunch Wraps

Preparation: 5 minutes **Cooking Time:** 10 minutes

Servings: 6

Ingredients:

- 6 wheat tostadas 2 c. sour cream

- 2 c. Mexican blend cheese 2 c. shredded lettuce

- 12 oz. low-sodium nacho cheese

- 3 Roma tomatoes 6 12-inch wheat tortillas

- 1 1/3 c. water 2 packets low-sodium taco seasoning

- 2 lbs. of lean ground beef

Directions:

1. Ensure your air fryer is preheated to 400°F.

2. Make beef according to taco seasoning packets.

3. Place 2/3 C. prepared beef, 4 tbsp. cheese, 1 tostada, 1/3 C. sour cream, 1/3 C. lettuce, 1/6th of tomatoes and 1/3 C. cheese on each tortilla.

4. Fold up tortillas edges and repeat with remaining ingredients.

5. Lay the folded sides of tortillas down into the air fryer and spray with olive oil.

6. Cook 2 minutes till browned.

Nutrition: Calories: 311 Fat: 9g Protein: 22g Sugar: 2g

18. Country Fried Steak

Preparation Time: 10 minutes

Cooking Time: 10 minutes

Servings: 2

Ingredients:

- 1 tsp. pepper

- 2 c. almond milk

- 2 tbsps. almond flour

- 6 oz. ground sausage meat

- 1 tsp. pepper

- 1 tsp. salt

- 1 tsp. garlic powder

- 1 tsp. onion powder

- 1 c. panko breadcrumbs

- 1 c. almond flour

- 3 beaten eggs

- 6 oz. sirloin steak, lbed till thin

Directions:

1. Season panko breadcrumbs with spices.

2. Dredge steak in flour, then egg, and then seasoned panko mixture.

3. Place into air fryer basket. Cook 12 minutes at 370°F.

4. To make sausage gravy, cook sausage and drain off fat, but reserve 2 tablespoons.

5. Add flour to sausage and mix until incorporated. Gradually mix in milk over medium to high heat till it becomes thick.

6. Season mixture with pepper and cook 3 minutes longer.

7. Serve steak topped with gravy and enjoy!

Nutrition: Calories: 395 Fat: 11g Protein: 39g Sugar: 5g

19. Tortilla ala Pork

Preparation Time: 10 minutes

Cooking Time: 16 minutes

Servings: 8

Ingredients:

- 1 juiced lime

- 10 whole wheat tortillas

- 2 ½ c. shredded mozzarella cheese

- 30 oz. of cooked and shredded pork tenderloin

Directions:

1. While preparing the Ingredients, ensure your air fryer

   is preheated to 380°F.

2. Drizzle pork with lime juice and gently mix.

3. Heat tortillas in the microwave with a moist paper towel to soften.

4. Add about 3 ounces of pork and ¼ cup of shredded cheese to each tortilla. Tightly roll them up.

5. Spray the Chefman air fryer basket with a bit of olive oil.

6. Air Fry. Set temperature to 380°F, and set time to 10 minutes. Air fry taquitos 7-10 minutes till tortillas turn a slight golden color, making sure to flip halfway through the cooking process.

Nutrition: Calories: 309; Fat: 11g. Protein:21g. Sugar:2g

20. Panko-Breaded Pork Chops

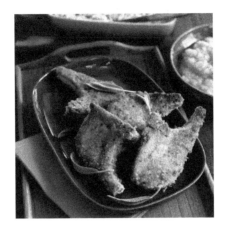

Preparation Time: 5 minutes

Cooking Time: 12 minutes

Servings: 6

Ingredients:

- 5 (3½- to 5-oz.) pork chops (bone-in or boneless)

- Seasoning salt

- Pepper

- ¼ cup all-purpose flour

- 2 tbsps. panko bread crumbs

- Cooking oil

Directions:

1. Prepare the Ingredients. Season the pork chops with the seasoning salt and pepper to taste.

2. Sprinkle the flour on both sides of the pork chops, then coat both sides with panko bread crumbs.

3. Place the pork chops in the air fryer. Stacking them is okay.

4. Spray the pork chops with cooking oil and air fry. Cook for 6 minutes.

5. Open the Chefman air fryer and flip the pork chops. Cook for an additional 6 minutes

6. Cool before serving.

7. Typically, bone-in pork chops are juicier than boneless. If you prefer really juicy pork chops, use bone-in.

Nutrition: Calories: 246; Fat: 13g. Protein: 26g. Fiber: 0g

Chapter 5 Poultry

21. Mexican Chicken

Preparation Time: 10 minutes

Cooking Time: 20 minutes

Servings: 4

Ingredients:

- 16 oz. salsa verde

- 1 tbsp. olive oil

- Salt and black pepper to the taste

- 1 lb chicken breast, boneless and skinless

- 1 and ½ cup Monterey Jack cheese, grated

- ¼ cup cilantro, chopped

- 1 tsp. garlic powder

Directions:

1. Pour salsa verde in a baking dish that fits your air fryer, season chicken with salt, pepper, garlic powder, brush with olive oil and place it over your salsa verde.

2. Introduce in your air fryer and cook at 380°F for 20 minutes.

3. Sprinkle cheese on top and cook for 2 minutes more.

4. Divide among plates and serve hot.

Nutrition: Calories 340 Fat 18g Fiber 14g Carbs 32g Protein 18g

22.   Honey Duck Breasts

Preparation Time: 10 minutes

Cooking Time: 22 minutes

Servings: 2

Ingredients:

- 1 smoked duck breast, halved

- 1 tsp. honey

- 1 tsp. tomato paste

- 1 tbsp. mustard ½ tsp. apple vinegar

Directions:

1. In a bowl, mix honey with tomato paste, mustard and

    vinegar; whisk well, add duck breast pieces, toss to

coat well, transfer to your air fryer and cook at 370°F for 15 minutes.

2. Take duck breast out of the fryer, add to the honey mix, toss again, return to air fryer and cook at 370°F for 6 minutes more.

3. Divide among plates and serve with a side salad.

Nutrition: Calories 274 Fat 11g Fiber 13g Carbs 22g Protein 13g

23. Roasted Chicken and Vegetable Salad

Preparation Time: 10 minutes

Cooking Time: 10 to 13 minutes

Servings: 4

Ingredients:

- 3 (4-oz./113-g.) low-sodium boneless, skinless chicken breasts, cut into 1-inch cubes

- 1 small red onion, sliced

- 1 red bell pepper, sliced

- 1 cup green beans, cut into 1-inch pieces

- 2 tbsps. low-fat ranch salad dressing

- 2 tbsps. freshly squeezed lemon juice

- ½ tsp. dried basil

- 4 cups mixed lettuce

Directions:

1. Preheat the air fryer to 400°F (204°C).

2. In the air fryer basket, roast the chicken, red onion, red bell pepper, and green beans for 10 to 13 minutes, or until the chicken reaches an internal temperature of 165°F (74°C) on a meat thermometer, tossing the food in the basket once during cooking.

3. While the chicken cooks, in a serving bowl, mix the ranch dressing, lemon juice, and basil.

4. Transfer the chicken and vegetables to a serving bowl and toss with the dressing to coat. Serve immediately on lettuce leaves.

Nutrition: Calories: 395 Fat: 11g Protein: 39g Sugar: 5g

24. Lemon Chicken and Spinach Salad

Preparation Time: 10 minutes

Cooking Time: 16 to 20 minutes

Servings: 4

Ingredients:

- 3 (5-oz./142-g.) low-sodium boneless, skinless chicken breasts, cut into 1-inch cubes

- 5 tsp.s olive oil

- ½ tsp. dried thyme

- 1 medium red onion, sliced

- 1 red bell pepper, sliced

- 1 small zucchini, cut into strips

- 3 tbsps. freshly squeezed lemon juice

- 6 cups fresh baby spinach

Directions:

1. Preheat the air fryer to 400°F (204°C).

2. In a large bowl, mix the chicken with olive oil and thyme. Toss to coat. Transfer to a medium metal bowl and roast for 8 minutes in the air fryer.

3. Add the red onion, red bell pepper, and zucchini. Roast for 8 to 12 minutes more, stirring once during cooking, or until the chicken reaches an internal temperature of 165°F (74°C) on a meat thermometer.

4. Remove the bowl from the air fryer and stir in the lemon juice.

5. Put the spinach in a serving bowl and top with the chicken mixture. Toss to combine and serve immediately.

Nutrition: Calories: 395 Fat: 11g Protein: 39g Sugar: 5g

25. Almond-Crusted Chicken Nuggets

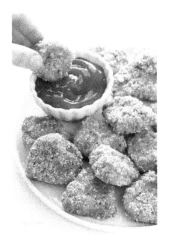

Preparation Time: 10 minutes

Cooking Time: 10 to 13 minutes

Servings: 4

Ingredients:

- 1 egg white

- 1 tbsp. freshly squeezed lemon juice

- ½ tsp. dried basil

- ½ tsp. ground paprika

- 1 lb. (454 g.) low-sodium boneless, skinless chicken breasts, cut into 1½-inch cubes

- ½ cup ground almonds

- 2 slices low-sodium whole-wheat bread, crumbled

Directions:

1. Preheat the air fryer to 400°F (204°C).

2. In a shallow bowl, beat the egg white, lemon juice, basil, and paprika with a fork until foamy.

3. Add the chicken and stir to coat.

4. On a plate, mix the almonds and bread crumbs.

5. Toss the chicken cubes in the almond and bread crumb mixture until coated.

6. Bake the nuggets in the air fryer, in two batches, for 10 to 13 minutes, or until the chicken reaches an internal temperature of 165°F (74°C) on a meat thermometer. Serve immediately.

Nutrition: Calories: 395 Fat: 11g Protein: 39g Sugar: 5g

26. Easy Tandoori Chicken

Preparation Time: 5 minutes

Cooking Time: 18 to 23 minutes

Servings: 4

Ingredients:

- 2/3 cup plain low-fat yogurt

- 2 tbsps. freshly squeezed lemon juice

- 2 tsps. curry powder

- ½ tsp. ground cinnamon

- 2 garlic cloves, minced

- 2 tsps. olive oil

- 4 (5-oz./142-g.) low-sodium boneless, skinless chicken breasts

Directions:

1. In a medium bowl, whisk the yogurt, lemon juice, curry powder, cinnamon, garlic, and olive oil.

2. With a sharp knife, cut thin slashes into the chicken. Add it to the yogurt mixture and turn to coat. Let stand for 10 minutes at room temperature. You can also prepare this ahead of time and marinate the chicken in the refrigerator for up to 24 hours.

3. Preheat the air fryer to 360°F (182°C).

4. Remove the chicken from the marinade and shake off any excess liquid. Discard any remaining marinade.

5. Roast the chicken for 10 minutes. With tongs, carefully turn each piece. Roast for 8 to 13 minutes more, or until the chicken reaches an internal temperature of 165°F (74°C) on a meat thermometer. Serve immediately.

Nutrition: Calories: 395 Fat: 11g Protein: 39g Sugar: 5g

Chapter 6 Fish & Seafood

27. Crab Cakes with Bell Peppers

Preparation Time: 5 minutes

Cooking Time: 10 minutes

Servings: 4

Ingredients:

- 8 oz. (227 g.) jumbo lump crab meat

- 1 egg, beaten

- Juice of ½ lemon

- 1/3 cup bread crumbs

- ¼ cup diced green bell pepper

- ¼ cup diced red bell pepper

- ¼ cup mayonnaise

- 1 tbsp. Old Bay seasoning

- 1 tsp. flour

- Cooking spray

Directions:

1. Press "Pre-Heat", set the temperature at 375°F (190°C).

2. Make the crab cakes: Place all the ingredients, except the flour and oil in a large bowl and stir until well incorporated.

3. Divide the crab mixture into four equal portions and shape each portion into a patty with your hands. Top

each patty with a sprinkle of ¼ teaspoon of flour.

4. Arrange the crab cakes in the air fryer basket and spray them with cooking spray.

5. Air fry for 10 minutes, flipping the crab cakes halfway through, or until they are cooked through.

6. Divide the crab cakes among four plates and serve.

Nutrition: Calories: 395 Fat: 11g Protein: 39g Sugar: 5g

28. Crab Cakes with Lettuce and Apple Salad

Preparation Time: 10 minutes

Cooking Time: 13 minutes

Servings: 2

Ingredients:

- 8 oz. (227 g.) lump crab meat, picked over for shells

- 2 tbsps. panko bread crumbs

- 1 scallion, minced

- 1 large egg

- 1 tbsp. mayonnaise

- 1½ tsps. dijon mustard

- Pinch of cayenne pepper

- 2 shallots, sliced thin

- 1 tbsp. extra-virgin olive oil, divided

- 1 tsp. lemon juice, plus lemon wedges for serving

- 1/8 tsp. salt

- Pinch of pepper

- ½ (3-oz./85-g.) small head Bibb lettuce, torn into bite-size pieces

- ½ apple, cored and sliced thin

Directions:

1. Press "Pre-Heat", set the temperature to 400°F (204°C).

2. Line large plate with triple layer of paper towels. Transfer crab meat to the prepared plate and pat dry with additional paper towels. Combine panko, scallion, egg, mayonnaise, mustard, and cayenne in a bowl. Using a rubber spatula, gently fold in crab meat until combined; discard paper towels. Divide crab mixture into 4 tightly packed balls, then flatten each into the 1-inch-thick cake (cakes will be delicate). Transfer cakes to plate and refrigerate until firm, about 10 minutes.

3. Toss shallots with ½ teaspoon oil in a separate bowl; transfer to air fryer basket. Air fry until shallots are browned, 5 to 7 minutes, tossing once halfway

through cooking. Return shallots to a now-empty bowl and set aside.

4. Arrange crab cakes in an air fryer basket, spaced evenly apart. Return basket to air fryer and air fry until crab cakes are light golden brown on both sides, 8 to 10 minutes, flipping and rotating cakes halfway through cooking.

5. Meanwhile, whisk the remaining 2½ teaspoons oil, lemon juice, salt, and pepper together in a large bowl. Add lettuce, apple, and shallots and toss to coat. Serve crab cakes with salad, passing lemon wedges separately.

Nutrition: Calories: 395 Fat: 11g Protein: 39g Sugar: 5g

29.   Crab Cakes with Sriracha Mayonnaise

Preparation Time: 15 minutes

Cooking Time: 10 minutes

Servings: 4

Ingredients:

Sriracha Mayonnaise:

- 1 cup mayonnaise

- 1 tbsp. sriracha

- 1½ tsps. freshly squeezed lemon juice

Crab Cakes:

- 1 tsp. extra-virgin olive oil

- ¼ cup finely diced red bell pepper

- ¼ cup diced onion

- ¼ cup diced celery

- 1 lb. (454 g.) lump crab meat

- 1 tsp. Old Bay seasoning

- 1 egg

- 1½ tsps. freshly squeezed lemon juice

- 1¾ cups panko bread crumbs, divided

- Vegetable oil, for spraying

Directions:

1. Mix the mayonnaise, sriracha, and lemon juice in a small bowl. Place 2/3 cup of the mixture in a separate bowl to form the base of the crab cakes. Cover the remaining sriracha mayonnaise and refrigerate. (This

will become dipping sauce for the crab cakes once they are cooked.)

2. Heat the olive oil in a heavy-bottomed, medium skillet over medium-high heat. Add the bell pepper, onion, and celery and sauté for 3 minutes. Transfer the vegetables to the bowl with the reserved 2/3 cup of sriracha mayonnaise. Mix in the crab, Old Bay seasoning, egg, and lemon juice. Add 1 cup of the panko. Form the crab mixture into 8 cakes. Dredge the cakes in the remaining ¾ cup of panko, turning to coat. Place on a baking sheet. Cover and refrigerate for at least 1 hour and up to 8 hours.

3. Press "Pre-Heat", set the temperature to 375°F (191°C). Spray the air fryer basket with oil. Working

in batches as needed so as not to overcrowd the basket, place the chilled crab cakes in a single layer in the basket. Spray the crab cakes with oil. Bake until golden brown, 8 to 10 minutes, carefully turning halfway through cooking. Remove to a platter and keep warm. Repeat with the remaining crab cakes as needed. Serve the crab cakes immediately with sriracha mayonnaise dipping sauce.

Nutrition: Calories: 395 Fat: 11g Protein: 39g Sugar: 5g

30. Crab Ratatouille with Eggplant and Tomatoes

Preparation Time: 15 minutes

Cooking Time: 11 to 14 minutes

Servings: 4

Ingredients:

- 1½ cups peeled and cubed eggplant

- 2 large tomatoes, chopped

- 1 red bell pepper, chopped

- 1 onion, chopped

- 1 tbsp. olive oil

- ½ tsp. dried basil

- ½ tsp. dried thyme

- Pinch salt

- Freshly ground black pepper, to taste

- 1½ cups cooked crab meat

Directions:

1. Press "Pre-Heat", set the temperature to 400°F (204°C).

2. In a metal bowl, stir together the eggplant, tomatoes, bell pepper, onion, olive oil, basil and thyme. Season with salt and pepper.

3. Place the bowl in the preheated air fryer and roast for 9 minutes.

4. Remove the bowl from the air fryer. Add the crab meat and stir well and roast for another 2 to 5 minutes, or until the vegetables are softened and the ratatouille is bubbling.

5. Serve warm.

Nutrition: Calories: 395 Fat: 11g Protein: 39g Sugar: 5g

31. Crawfish Creole Casserole

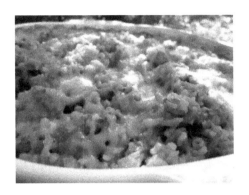

Preparation Time: 20 minutes

Cooking Time: 25 minutes

Servings: 4

Ingredients:

- 1½ cups crawfish meat

- ½ cup chopped celery

- ½ cup chopped onion

- ½ cup chopped green bell pepper

- 2 large eggs, beaten

- 1 cup half-and-half

- 1 tbsp. butter, melted

- 1 tbsp. cornstarch

- 1 tsp. Creole seasoning

- ¾ tsp. salt

- ½ tsp. freshly ground black pepper

- 1 cup shredded Cheddar cheese

- Cooking spray

Directions:

1. In a medium bowl, stir together the crawfish, celery, onion, and green pepper.

2. In another medium bowl, whisk the eggs, half-and-half, butter, cornstarch, Creole seasoning, salt, and pepper until blended. Stir the egg mixture into the crawfish mixture. Add the cheese and stir to combine.

3. Press "Pre-Heat", set the temperature at 300°F (149°C). Spray a baking pan with oil.

4. Transfer the crawfish mixture to the prepared pan and place it in the air fryer basket.

5. Bake for 25 minutes, stirring every 10 minutes, until a knife inserted into the center comes out clean.

6. Serve immediately.

Nutrition: Calories: 395 Fat: 11g Protein: 39g Sugar: 5g

32. Crab Cakes

Preparation Time: 5 minutes

Cooking Time: 10 minutes

Servings: 4

Ingredients:

- 8 oz. jumbo lump crabmeat

- 1 tbsp. Old Bay Seasoning

- 1/3 cup bread crumbs

- ¼ cup diced red bell pepper

- ¼ cup diced green bell pepper

- 1 egg ¼ cup mayonnaise

- Juice of ½ lemon 1 tsp. flour Cooking oil

Directions:

1. In a large bowl, combine the crabmeat, Old Bay Seasoning, bread crumbs, red bell pepper, green bell pepper, egg, mayo, and lemon juice. Mix gently to combine.

2. Form the mixture into 4 patties. Sprinkle ¼ teaspoon of flour on top of each patty.

3. Place the crab cakes in the air fryer. Spray them with cooking oil. Cook for 10 minutes.

4. Serve.

Nutrition: Calories: 176; Total fat: 8g. Saturated fat: 1g. Cholesterol: 101mg. Sodium: 826mg. Carbohydrates: 12g. Fiber: 1g. Protein: 15g

33.   Coconut Shrimp

Preparation Time: 10 minutes

Cooking Time: 10 minutes

Servings: 4

Ingredients:

- 1 lb. raw shrimp, peeled and deveined (see Prep tip, here)

- 1 egg

- ¼ cup all-purpose flour

- 1/3 cup shredded unsweetened coconut

- ¼ cup panko bread crumbs

- Salt

- Pepper

- Cooking oil

Directions:

1. Dry the shrimp with paper towels.

2. In a small bowl, beat the egg. In another small bowl, place the flour. In a third small bowl, combine the coconut and panko bread crumbs, and season with salt and pepper to taste. Mix well.

3. Spray the air fryer basket with cooking oil.

4. Dip the shrimp in the flour, then the egg, and then the coconut and bread crumb mixture.

5. Place the shrimp in the air fryer. It is okay to stack them. Cook for 4 minutes.

6. Open the air fryer and flip the shrimp. I recommend flipping individually instead of shaking, which keeps the breading intact. Cook for an additional 4 minutes or until crisp.

7. Cool before serving.

Nutrition: Calories: 182; Total fat: 6g. Saturated fat: 3g. Cholesterol: 246mg. Sodium: 780mg. Carbohydrates: 8g. Fiber: 1g. Protein: 24g

Chapter 7 Vegetables

34. Indian Turnips Salad

Preparation Time: 10 minutes

Cooking Time: 12 minutes

Servings: 4

Ingredients:

- 20 oz. turnips, peeled and chopped

- 1 tsp. garlic, minced

- 1 tsp. ginger, grated

- 2 yellow onions, chopped

- 2 tomatoes, chopped

- 1 tsp. cumin, ground

- 1 tsp. coriander, ground

- 2 green chilies, chopped

- ½ tsp. turmeric powder

- 2 tbsps. butter

- Salt and black pepper to the taste

- A handful of coriander leaves, chopped

Directions:

1. Heat a pan that fits your air fryer with the butter, melt it, add green chilies, garlic and ginger, stir and cook for 1 minute.

2. Add onions, salt, pepper, tomatoes, turmeric, cumin, ground coriander and turnips, stir, introduce in your air fryer and cook at 350°F for 10 minutes.

3. Divide among plates, sprinkle fresh coriander on top, and serve.

4. Enjoy!

Nutrition: Calories 100, Fat 3g. Fiber 6g. Carbs 12g. Protein 4g

35. Spinach Pie

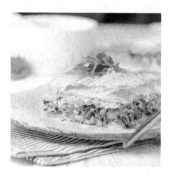

Preparation Time: 10 minutes

Cooking Time: 15 minutes

Servings: 4

Ingredients:

- 7 oz. flour

- 2 tbsps. butter

- 7 oz. spinach

- 1 tbsp. olive oil

- 2 eggs

- 2 tbsps. milk

- 3 oz. cottage cheese

- Salt and black pepper to the taste

- 1 yellow onion, chopped

Directions:

1. In your food processor, mix flour with butter, 1 egg, milk, salt and pepper, blend well, transfer to a bowl, knead, cover, and leave for 10 minutes.

2. Heat a pan with the oil over medium-high heat, add onion and spinach, stir and cook for 2 minutes.

3. Add salt, pepper, the remaining egg and cottage cheese, stir well and take off the heat.

4. Divide dough into 4 pieces, roll each piece, place on the bottom of a ramekin, add spinach filling over dough, place ramekins in your air fryer's basket, and cook at 360°F for 15 minutes.

5. Serve warm,

6. Enjoy!

Nutrition: Calories 250, Fat 12g. Fiber 2g. Carbs 23g. Protein 12g

36.   Beets and Blue Cheese Salad

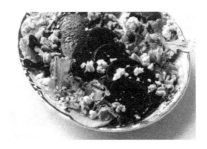

Preparation Time: 10 minutes

Cooking Time: 14 minutes

Servings: 6

Ingredients:

- 6 beets, peeled and quartered

- Salt and black pepper to the taste

- ¼ cup blue cheese, crumbled

- 1 tbsp. olive oil

Directions:

1. Put beets in your air fryer, cook them at 350°F for 14 minutes and transfer them to a bowl.

2. Add blue cheese, salt, pepper and oil, toss and serve.

3. Enjoy!

Nutrition: Calories 100, Fat 4g. Fiber 4g. Carbs 10g. Protein 5g

Chapter 8 Side Dish

37. Brussels Sprouts Side Dish

Preparation Time: 15 minutes

Cooking Time: 20 minutes

Servings: 5

Ingredients:

- 3 tbsps. roasted garlic, crushed

- 1 cup mayonnaise

- 1 tsp. thyme, chopped

- 8 tsps. olive oil

- Salt and black pepper according to your taste

- 2 lbs. Brussels sprouts, trimmed and halved

Directions:

1. Combine the Brussels sprouts with pepper, salt, and oil in your air fryer, mix properly, and sear for about 15 minutes at around 390°F.

2. In the meantime, blend thyme with garlic and mayo in a bowl and blend well.

3. Brussels sprouts are placed on bowls; garlic sauce is drizzled all over and eaten as a side dish. Enjoy!

Nutrition: Calories: 395 Fat: 11g Protein: 39g Sugar: 5g

38. Herbed Potatoes

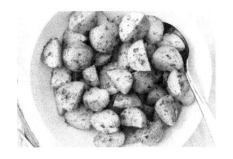

Preparation Time: 15 minutes

Cooking Time: 25 minutes

Servings: 5

Ingredients:

- A pinch of cinnamon powder

- A pinch of ginger powder

- 1 tsp. cumin, ground

- 4 tbsps. mayonnaise

- ½ cup ketchup

- ½ tsp. coriander, ground

- 1 tsp. curry powder

- 4 tbsps. olive oil

- Salt and black pepper according to your taste

- 4 sweet potatoes, peeled and cut into medium fries

Directions:

1. Mix the sweet potato fries with pepper, salt, curry powder, coriander, and oil in your air fryer's basket, mix well and steam for about 20 minutes at around 370°F, turning once.

2. Meanwhile, blend the ginger, cumin, mayo, and cinnamon with some ketchup in a container and stir well.

3. On bowls, split fries, drizzle ketchup blend over them and eat as a side dish. Enjoy!

Nutrition: Calories: 395 Fat: 11g Protein: 39g Sugar: 5g

Chapter 9 Appetizers

39. Italian Shrimp Platter

Preparation Time: 5 minutes

Cooking Time: 12 minutes

Servings: 4

Ingredients:

- 1 lb. shrimp, peeled and deveined

- 1 tbsp. Italian seasoning

- ½ tsp. cumin, ground

- ½ tsp. mustard seeds, crushed

- 2 tbsps. lemon juice

- Salt and black pepper to the taste

- A drizzle of olive oil

Directions:

1. In the air fryer's basket, combine the shrimp with the seasoning and the other ingredients, toss and cook at 390°F for 12 minutes flipping them halfway.

2. Arrange the shrimp on a platter and serve as an appetizer.

Nutrition: Calories 200, Fat 5g. Fiber 3g. Carbs 13g. Protein 4g

40. Potato Chips in Chili

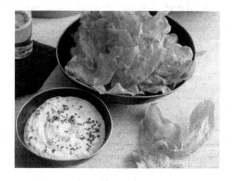

Preparation Time: 10 minutes

Cooking Time: 20 minutes

Servings: 4

Ingredients:

- 2 sweet potatoes, thinly sliced

- 1 tsp. sweet paprika

- 1 tsp. chili powder

- Salt and black pepper to the taste

- 1 tbsp. olive oil

Directions:

1. In your air fryer's basket, mix the potato chips with the paprika and the other ingredients, toss and cook at 400°F for 20 minutes, flipping them halfway.

2. Serve as a snack.

Nutrition: Calories 143, Fat 4g. Fiber 1.5g. Carbs 10g. Protein 5g

Conclusion

<u>We have reached the end of our journey and I remind you that now is your time! Leave a review with a photo of a dish cooked using this cookbook and accept the challenge!</u>

Can you cook like Brandon?

Air fryers turn flavorful fresh ingredients into delicious dishes with less oil than deep frying. I would highly recommend this book to anyone who loves cooking and is always looking for new foods to try. It's a cookbook that doesn't require a lot of time or ingredients to create some amazing dishes! The examples in this cookbook are quite diverse which proves that you can make almost anything using an air fryer, from snacks like mozzarella sticks and French fries, over pastries like doughnuts and croissants, all the way to main courses like steak or lamb chops. The recipes in this book range from simple to elaborate but I would say that they all look delicious.

The book is not written in the typical cookbook way where it only tells you how to do something but rather it includes a couple of pictures that will help you understand what the finished product will look like. If there is anything I think this book needs, it would be more recipes that are simple enough for my mom to make. Most of the recipes included here require special ingredients or some cooking skills and will likely turn out better if your family has the necessary skills already. I think this book should be advertised as being a guide for people who have air fryers already and have some cooking abilities.

The recipes included here will help you get the most out of your air fryer. I'm always interested in getting new appliances but I don't like to waste my money on things that I won't be able to use. If I were to buy an air fryer, I would definitely pick up this book first. The recipes included here are all you need to make delicious meals and snacks with your air fryer. You really can't go wrong with this book!

If you're new to air frying, or simply want to learn more about it, I would highly recommend this book for your first step. Yes, there are many recipes included here that may be hard for a beginner to make but there's also quite a few that will prove easy and make your next dinner party one to remember. Lots of wonderful recipes are included here.

Possible dislikes: Nothing much, if I had to list down something, it would be more recipes requiring less ingredients or that are easier for beginners to make but that's an easy fix and the author should have made some catering options for specific events. If you're looking to add a little more flavor into your cooking, you'll love this book!

CPSIA information can be obtained
at www.ICGtesting.com
Printed in the USA
BVHW041408220621
610211BV00005B/1475

9 781911 685234